HOW YOU CAN
DRINK
MORE
WATER
EVERY DAY

ERIC FOSTER

TABLE OF **CONTENTS**

FOREWORD

This isn't a just book about water. You won't find a section titled "13 Health Benefits of Drinking More Water" like some transported and overpriced blog post. This is a book about how to get your head on straight so you can start creating habits that stick for life. At least, that's what it aspires to.

It's also a personal book. If you don't care to read about the time I almost puked on a little girl, this book isn't for you. And if you want statistics and hard science about water—again, this is the wrong book. I assume you're smart enough to find facts like that on Google. So while I hope this book educates you, I also wrote it to entertain you. At least, that's what I aspired to.

Eric Foster

August 10, 2016

INTRODUCTION

A year ago today, I joined a health and fitness program. One of the first challenges was to drink three liters of water a day for five of the next seven days. That's six standard 500ml bottles of water, just under 13 cups—104 ounces a day.

We all know drinking more water is healthy, but compared to the usual recommendation—eight eight-ounce glasses a day—that sounded like a devastating amount of water.

But I had already joined the program and I was up for the challenge. So I decided to up the ante a bit: Instead of any five days out of the following week, I would do five in a row. To track my progress, I scrawled thirty checkboxes on an index card, six for each day, and stuck it to the back of my bedroom door.

Bottle down, X on the card, a little celebration, and I could see myself making progress.

But it wasn't all peachy in waterland.

The first few days, I failed to account for everything else I was drinking. My drink of choice at the time was unsweetened tea with a wedge of lemon, and that remained my go-to option—at least until the third day.

After a three days guzzling down liter upon liter of water—in addition to countless glasses of iced tea—my stomach felt like it would burst. So I was an idiot, attacking the challenge with no deeper strategy than *you're not allowed to sleep until you drink the damn water.* And on day four, feeling bloated and slightly awful, I cut back on the tea.

But the rest of my strategy didn't change much. So there I was, ten o'clock the next night, throwing back a liter and a half of water and drawing tiny X's on my doorframe.

Because *you're not allowed to sleep until you drink the damn water.*

Yeah. Like I was going to sleep after drinking a liter and a half of water.

But I made it to day five, my insides maybe a little too moistened, and barreled through the final day on water alone. But even with a workout and a walk in the August sun, three liters still felt like overkill.

And that evening, ready to bang a nail in the challenge's coffin, I chugged the day's final liter. Then—with the same belt-loosening pride I imagine courses through veins of a competitive eater after swallowing 35 hot dogs—I crushed the empty Dasani bottle, threw it in the trash, and swore I would never drink water again.

So, obviously, I have no idea what I'm doing. But after slaying the hydra and retreating to the safety and comfort of iced tea, I still wanted to drink more water than I had in the past. Not three liters a day, but maybe two, just over the standard 64-ounce recommendation. That seemed doable.

Still, there were obstacles. If you've ever considered boosting your water intake but kept running into problems, finding excuses, or just weren't sure where to start, maybe some of these objections sound familiar:

- I'll get bored drinking plain water all the time.
- I don't want to give up my beer, coffee, or soda.
- If I drink that much water, I'll have to pee all day.

Throughout the rest of this book, I've put together actionable strategies you can use to get over your hurdles, get healthy, and drink more water. Plus, we'll discuss several stupid water myths that keep getting passed around as folk wisdom along with a few unconventional thoughts about how drinking more water can improve not only your physical life, but your mental and emotional resilience as well.

If you need specific tactics for increasing your water intake or making fewer unhealthy choices, that's covered too. But first, to guide you through your journey towards drinking more water, I organized the book around a loose framework with the appallingly cute name of the **O.A.S.I.S. Method**. More on that on the next page.

1

THE O.A.S.I.S. METHOD

It amuses me how some authors stretch definitions and search out synonyms just to wrap their ideas in something cool, catchy, and marketable. The worse the synonyms, the further the stretch, the more amusing it is. And in light of that, I told myself if I ever wrote a self-help book, I would cram the advice into the framework of a clumsy acronym.

So I'd like to introduce you to the **O.A.S.I.S. Method**. The **O.A.S.I.S. Method** is *my* cutesy, ham-fisted acronym, and I've wrapped it around the structure of an otherwise sensible if circumlocutious and rather irreverent book. It comprises the following five steps:

1. OVERCOME obstacles and myths

The first step in habit change of any sort is to understand the landscape. Almost every topic— fitness, business, romance, etc.—is drenched in lies, half-truths, and bad advice. Not only that, but there are always personal obstacles that get in our way. Those obstacles can be mental or physical, real or imagined, but we must overcome them before we can get started improving our lives.

Maybe you don't like the taste of plain water. Maybe you don't want to give up caffeine. Maybe you can't afford bottled water or a water filter.

All of those challenges can be overcome. But we have to be brutally honest with ourselves and consciously decide to overcome them. Then, we need to know how to overcome them. And, finally, we need to commit to overcoming them.

Until we get the lay of the land and establish a strategy for overcoming the obstacles we face, our attempts at behavior change remain futile. Problems will take us by surprise. The unexpected will attack. And, most likely, we'll give up.

This is why most diets and workout plans fail. What do you do when you really want a cookie? What happens when life gets hectic? What happens if you come down sick and miss the gym a few weeks in a row? If you don't have a system in place that helps you over these rough spots, it's easy to get derailed.

So the first things we need to do are learn the landscape, figure out the deep reason why we want to drink more water, and discover what's stopping us from doing it already.

Once we've done that, we can acknowledge our current habits and accept where we're starting from.

2. ACKNOWLEDGE current habits

Wherever we are, we need to accept it. Lying to ourselves only hurts us in the end.

If you haven't had a sip of plain water in over a decade, that's not a moral failure. But if you haven't had a sip in over a decade and still tell yourself that you drink water "sometimes"? That might be.

Whether you want to shed the cappuccinos and Coke for effortless weight loss or you're just looking to slip a few more cups of water into your day, knowing where you're coming from is crucial.

When we know what our starting point really is, it becomes easy to measure progress and acknowledge setbacks. When we're familiar with our current habits, we can track the changes we make to them. And when we track the changes, it's harder to lie to ourselves and easier to see how far we've come. If we don't know where we're starting from, success can look like failure—or worse, we can trick ourselves into calling failure a success.

3. START changing bad habits

Once we know what our habits are, it's time to start changing them. The hardest part about changing habits is that we don't know what will work until we test it. A plan that helped someone else quit smoking might have us back to a pack a day within a week.

So when we try to improve our habits, we have to have the mindset of a scientist and an attitude of experimentation. Every change we make is only a test. It might work, or it might not. But the outcome of any single experiment doesn't matter. What matters is that we learn something from trying. And when something doesn't work, we try something else. And we keep trying until we find what works.

Why is changing our habits so hard? Because even if we know what they are, we probably don't know the deeper reason of *why* they are. We only develop habits because we're getting some benefit from them, and the real benefit is rarely obvious. You might need your afternoon coffee for energy— or it might just be a chance to get up from your desk. And those three beers every Friday night could only be an excuse to hang out with your friends; maybe you'd be just as happy trading each pint for a glass of water.

Until you experiment and figure out what new behavior fills the same need as the old undesirable one, new and improved habits won't stick.

4. INCREASE water intake

Increasing your water intake may coincide with changing bad habits. You may choose to replace certain beverages with water. But you may not. Such a drastic change can be difficult and discouraging. Swapping in water when you really want soda could be a step too far.

Even so, if you want to drink more water, you'll have to make baby steps towards your long-term goal. At first, you might call it a victory if you stop yourself from pouring that second cup of coffee or switching out regular soda for diet. In the beginning stages of behavior change and habit creation, the endgame—becoming the type of person who drinks water—matters less than the process of learning how to get there.

So when we make small changes, we might not end up drinking more water right away. At some point, though, we will figure out where we can fit water into our lives. It might be as a replacement for something we used to drink, or it might be an addition, such as drinking a glass of water first thing in the morning.

But always keep in mind that small changes count just as much if not more than overnight resolutions. As most people can attest every year in early February, big resolutions beget failure—it's almost clockwork. So one extra glass of water a day is worth celebrating. And going from three cups of coffee to two is a win, even if you're trying to kick the caffeine habit altogether.

Once we've started changing our habits and increasing our water intake, we can track our new behaviors. And then we're able to study the results to find insights and see which changes are working and which ones aren't.

5. STUDY the results

Here's the moment of truth. Are you reducing or replacing your bad habits? Are you drinking more water?

After you've made a few experiments and tracked the results, you can go back and study them weeks or months later to see if you achieved and maintained the desired outcome.

Without measuring what you've been doing, it's hard to know if you've made a lasting change. Maybe you feel like you're drinking a lot of water, but you're not actually drinking it as often as you'd like. Or you're drinking it erratically—you're trying, but it's still neither a habit nor your default beverage choice. Or maybe you surpassed your goal and have had nothing but water to drink for the past two months.

You won't know unless you're keeping track. And once you know, you can make adjustments to fix things that aren't working or to improve even further.

That's the **O.A.S.I.S. Method** in a nutshell. The book wends its way around this five point framework without adhering to it religiously. At the end, I'll tie everything back together and give you a solid plan for increasing your water intake.

But first, let's talk about common obstacles to drinking more water.

2

OBSTACLES, OBJECTIONS, AND EXCUSES

I believe most of us, deep down, know exactly what we need to do to hit our goals. But we're also human. We're weak. It's easy for us to make excuses, ignore advice, and generally sit around with our thumbs up our asses.

What's hard is buckling down and being brutally honest. Not many of us are able to be honest with ourselves, because when we look in the mirror, a lot of time we don't like what we see.

We're not perfect. We're not living up to our potential. We're not good enough. We fail, we fuck up, we get rejected—all the time. But that's okay. That's what makes us human. It's what makes us interesting. *Everything went right and they lived happily after* is a bad story that no one wants to hear.

So whether you're trying to get a promotion, raise a decent kid, or simply drink more water, your challenge starts with getting your mindset right.

And to start, you need to approach your goal-setting with total, guilt-free honesty about what your priorities are and what's really holding you back.

Here are the most common obstacles, excuses, and objections people have for not drinking more water. I can't see inside your brain, so you may have other things going on, but this list will at least stir up the barriers in your own mind and help you find ways to fit more water into your life.

1. I don't like the taste of water.

I used to drink all of my water with lemon juice—massive amounts of it. I would buy giant bottles of lemon juice from the store because I just couldn't afford enough real, fresh lemons to keep up with my habit. I'd even buy several bottles at time because the thought of running out was unfathomable.

But every few months, I would screw up. At 11pm, after all the stores were closed, I would open the fridge and find a couple of drops at the bottom of my last bottle. And that meant it was going to be one of those long, lemon juice free nights. I would be frustrated and upset for hours until I made it to the store the next day.

Looking back, it seems so silly. But I get it. Water's boring. If you're used to juice, soft drinks, lattes or whatever, switching to a flavorless liquid won't be easy.

But you can find a simple solution to ease the transition. Like me, you can flavor your water. Lemon juice was always my drug of choice, but limes are pretty cool, and I hear you can do some good work with mint, cucumber, ginger or rose petals.

Non-caffeinated, unsweetened herbal teas are also an option. Chamomile and rooibos are popular choices, and I've always been a fan of Tangerine Orange Zinger from Celestial Seasonings.

Another excellent idea is using a dash or two of bitters. With the rebirth of cocktail culture, you can find plenty of flavors online. The most popular brands include Angostura, Peychaud's, Regan's No. 6. While most bitters are alcoholic, don't worry about it. You only need a few drops. But if you want to avoid booze altogether, Fee Brothers makes a line of non-alcoholic bitters.

Aside from those tips, I'm not yet an expert on flavoring water. But to help you out, I put together a short guide called *5 Fast Flavored Water Recipes* that details a few of my favorite infused waters.

You can pick your copy up for free at www.esfoster.com/5fastwaters.

But in the end I feel that only drinking flavored water can be a crutch. It's not a bad crutch, especially if it helps you get more water in your system, but running out of tea or fruit while you still don't like plain water is an easy way to derail yourself from your goals.

If you want to make drinking water a robust habit that can't be thrown off by a little inconvenience, learn to drink water plain. It doesn't have to be difficult. You can start with flavored water and decrease the amount of your chosen flavoring agent until you wean yourself on the taste of plain water. That's a totally legit option. Even with my love of iced tea, for almost the past year I've brewed a gallon of tea using only four to six teabags and I rarely notice the difference.

2. Bottled water and water filters are expensive.

I paid 99 cents for a song called "Crying These Cocksucking Tears." Dasani costs 20 cents a bottle.

I like Dasani. I like that Coca-Cola figured out how to make a bottle that's sturdy but still good for the environment. They say it uses less plastic. It has a green leaf and a recycling triangle on the label.

Aquafina says their bottles are good for the environment too. They crinkle when you pick them up. If you suck out all the water, there's no integrity left. Less plastic, but no integrity. What's the point in being environmentally-friendly if you have no integrity?

The point is, either Coke is lying or Pepsi is stupid.

3. My tap water tastes bad.

I drink bottled water because I think my tap water tastes funny. Almost no one else notices it. I cook with it. I make tea with it. I brush my teeth with it. But I swear it tastes funny. Maybe I just want to feel special.

But I don't feel special. I feel like I should suck it up and drink tap water.

I just got myself a glass straight from the faucet.

Nassim Taleb wrote a book called *Antifragile*. It's about things that get better through disorder. I haven't read it. I read the cover and the Amazon reviews. But I get the idea that drinking only bottled water is a kind of fragility. Like refusing to leave the house because my chihuahua's tutu is in the wash.

And the Stoics had this idea where they practiced hardship so they wouldn't suffer as much when things actually got hard. I picture the Romans drinking tap water once a week instead of Evian or Fiji.

Modern technology lets me shoot water through holes in my house. When I think about that, I'm almost in awe. So instead of waiting for the tutu to dry, I'm going to go ahead and drink this glass of water.

If I die, you'll never read this.

4. Tap water is dangerous.

Everyday we get in cars and relationships and cell phone contracts.

You're going to die in a car accident next week. Your boyfriend will smack you in the head and sleep with your sister and you'll have to poison him. You probably can't get a signal inside your own home.

Lots of things are dangerous. If you live your life from calamity to calamity, you'll end up in Snowflake, Arizona, allergic to oxygen and thinking you can smell electricity.

5. Won't all this water make me pee a lot?

I'm writing this on the toilet. I do some of my best work on the toilet.

The science seems to say that your body will accustom itself to an increased water intake. So you might pee a lot for a few days. That's your body saying, "Mmm, delicious magic." It's your body thanking you for giving it water. Your body is 75% water, so it needs a lot.

If you think peeing a lot is bad, don't drink extra water. Just drink it instead of what you usually drink. And if it turns out water makes you pee forever, get a laptop and a cell phone. You can work on the toilet.

6. I'm not giving up my coffee, soda, beer, etc.

We already talked about becoming antifragile and Romans drinking tap water. That applies here too. If I can't go without some drug, I feel terrible. You don't need drugs to have a good time.

CAFFEINE

Caffeine won't kill you, but in most cases it's unnecessary. If I need coffee or tea or go pills to get up in the morning, it means I'm doing something wrong. Probably sleep. It probably means I should sleep more.

I heard somewhere the US loses two billion dollars a year in productivity because of sleep deprivation. I don't know the actual number.

Think about that. Businesses could make millions of dollars if their employees didn't come to work on time.

SUGAR

Sugar will kill you.

The Canadians made a compelling documentary called *Sugar Coated* you can watch on Netflix. The sugar industry is following the tobacco playbook: Create doubt and plausible deniability so you can't be held responsible. Commission studies. Win public relations awards.

And it's worse because it's sugar. Sugar is everywhere and in everything. We eat sugar when we're happy. We eat it when we're sad. We eat it when we're bored. We even put sugar in things that don't taste sweet and eat them too.

We're all going to die.

ALCOHOL

One time I went to an AA picnic with a friend. Someone asked me where I was from. I answered him and asked the same question. Then he told me. That was the whole conversation. There may have been a nod at the end. I'm not an impressive conversationalist.

But I enjoyed the stories the speakers told. They all had the same story:

I did drugs and drank and had sex and it was bad. Then I found AA and I did more drugs and drank and had sex and it was bad. Then I found AA again and I worked the steps and I really tried this time and then God touched me in my happy place and now I'm not doing drugs or drinking or having sex and it is good.

They didn't say anything about water. But I guess if you give up drugs and alcohol and sex, water could be the most exciting part of your day.

Maybe some of them were baptized.

Maybe you do need drugs to have a good time.

3

STUPID WATER MYTHS

When I decided to write this book, I started researching facts and myths about water and dehydration, food and exercise, all sorts of things. What I realized is I don't know anything. Neither does anyone else. We're just all struggling along passing on the latest gossip and passing off the strangest factoid.

Will drinking more water improve your skin? Will caffeinated beverages dehydrate you? Does feeling thirsty mean you're already dehydrated? Google says yes, no, and "it's complicated" to all those questions. And that's just page one.

So the theme of this chapter is *everyone is full of shit*. Including me. I have no idea what I'm doing. On the TV series *An Idiot Abroad*, Karl Pilkington announces that if he had a superpower, he'd be Bullshit Man. He would fly into office meetings and car dealerships, point his finger, and say, "That's bullshit!" As you read this chapter, imagine Bullshit Man standing over your shoulder.

1. You need to drink eight eight-ounce glasses of water a day.

If I was a better conspiracy theorist, I'd tell you everyone is lying to you. But I don't think that's the case. I think someone somewhere is making shit up, and everyone else is just passing turds down the line.

Maybe you've heard that you should walk at least 10,000 steps a day. And maybe you should. I don't know. It probably won't hurt. But who came up with the number 10,000? Certainly, there's a study somewhere. Or at least a fable. Maybe Goldilocks walked 10,000 steps a day.

The real origin of the number isn't much better. In 1965, a Japanese researcher showed that most people get less than 5,000 steps a day. He concluded that people would be healthier if they walked twice as much. So he began selling a pedometer called a *manpo-kei*, which is Japanese for "10,000 step meter." The round number was good marketing. Everyone repeated the 10,000 step claim until it became common knowledge.

But I feel sorry for lazy people with dreams. They buy a pedometer and only count 2,000 steps a day. Discouraged, they give up, chuck the pedometer in the back of a drawer and keep walking 2,000 steps a day. They think they'll never get to 10,000, so why bother. But 2,001 would have been a victory.

It's much the same with the common advice to drink eight glasses of water a day. It's not a bad goal, but it's a only an estimate. Everyone has varying needs for their water intake, and the truth is no one agrees about how much water we should be drinking.

Some argue 64 ounces is too much. Others say it's too little. Some say men and women have different needs, with women needing about two liters and men needing about three. The highest number I found was 3.8 liters. That recommendation was for pregnant women. I always thought it was the baby, but maybe all that water is why they look like they're about to explode.

What's the best target for you? I don't know. It's hard to tell. If you don't drink any water right now, start with a glass a day. Maybe half a glass. Maybe just a sip. Consider it your 2,001st step.

2. Only plain water counts towards your daily water intake goal.

There are people who only drink Coca-Cola. I saw them on the news. Or Dr. Phil. Or somewhere.

They're usually big people. I don't know how they fit through doors. They don't look like they'd fit through my door.

They say, "My family doesn't know. I hide all my snacks." Their family knows.

So they eat snacks and drink Coke and go on TV. So you can get all the water you need from snacks and Coke and TV.

But don't. You won't fit through doors.

3. Not drinking enough water isn't a big deal.

She wanted a black dog. So in the 95 degree heat, wearing a red dress shirt, black Dockers, and a patterned vest stolen from a tacky wizard, I pumped up a long balloon.

I was already feeling sick and half dizzy. Sweat hadn't stopped bleeding from my face since I clicked the A/C off in the car thirty minutes earlier. With every lull in the foot traffic, I took a knee and guzzled a bottle of water.

I was dying. Quite literally, dying—my body rebels in the heat. Forget the ridiculous outfit, the layers, and the dress shoes with long socks—even in beachwear, sweat stains my blonde hair brown and my stomach churns.

The latex squeaked as I twisted the dog's the head into shape, his airy little brain unable to conceive how traumatic the next five seconds in his short balloon life were going to be.

As I remember it (and this was at least eight years ago in the fog and delirium of the summer heat, so I may have invented the whole story for dramatic effect), the dog had one pair of legs when I vomited all over everything—my shirt, my hands, Chase Bank's advertising.

Thankfully, I missed the nine-year-old girl by a few inches. I dropped to the ground, trading my disabled dog for a bottle of water and gulped it down in a futile effort to quell my stomach. I continued to puke violently.

I clambered to my feet and went to find a trash can to aim for, rockets of vomit projecting from my mouth as I walked. I like to imagine I looked like the little girl from *The Exorcist* staggering through a park and spraying pea soup in every direction. I made it to the trash can, collapsed, and woke up in a hospital.

The first time anything like that happened, I was six years old. I only remember it in broken snapshots—puking in the toilet in the middle of the night, someone carrying me to the car. It was awful. Terrifying. And though my experience is on the outlying edge of dehydration symptoms, it demonstrates just how serious the issue can become. Add in a little heat and a little sweat, and you're fermenting disaster like a fine home brew.

Aside from serious complications like heat exhaustion, even mild dehydration can damage your body and diminish your performance. Some common symptoms of mild dehydration are fatigue, headaches, and anxiety.

Your school or work life can also be compromised. Dehydration has a negative impact on memory, mood, and concentration. It also slashes your reaction time, so driving dehydrated can put you at almost as much risk of a car accident as getting behind the wheel drunk or half asleep.

4. If you're thirsty, you're already dehydrated.

No, you're not. That's not how anything works. If it was, your stomach growling would mean you're starving to death and a stubbed toe would be reason to amputate. Probably at the knee.

5. Caffeinated beverages dehydrate you.

Beverages are mostly water. Caffeine makes you pee (and poop). I'm not a doctor.

You'll probably pee less water than you drank. You probably shouldn't chug gallons of coffee. I think that's what a doctor would say.

If you're really worried about it, he might give you Klonopin. I don't know. I'm not a doctor.

6. You need sports drinks when you exercise.

Exercise is hard. Drink something that makes you happy.

But if you want to lose weight, don't drink calories. Your fat cells are like stray cats. If you feed them, you'll never get rid of them.

Athletes have different needs. I don't know what they are. I'm not an athlete. You should find out before becoming an athlete.

7. You can drink too much water.

Water kills a lot of people. Most of them drown. Some of them drink too much water. But most of them drown.

Several years ago, a woman died after drinking two gallons in three hours without going to the bathroom. She was trying to win a Nintendo Wii. I don't know if she won.

I had trouble drinking six bottles a day. It made my stomach hurt.

Don't drink until your stomach hurts.

8. Drinking extra water will improve your skin.

Most of the internet says water will improve your skin. I guess that's what most women's magazines would say too.

The New York Times says it won't. They cited a scientist who said no one knows how water intake affects health or disease or general wellbeing.

The New York Times is a total buzzkill. For dry skin, they recommended moisturizer.

9. Water will help you detox.

When I quit smoking years ago, a gray film would seep out of my pores when I took a shower. This happened for weeks. It was disgusting.

But in most cases, anyone who's selling you on a detox is doing just that—selling you. Juice cleanse, master cleanse, magic pills—it's all a bunch of overpriced, ineffective nonsense.

The idea of a detox implies there are toxins in your body that you need to remove, but no one ever explains what those toxins actually are. It's just a vague notion of something ominous.

So if you're ever considering buying a detox, ask which toxins are in your body, how the salesman diagnosed you, and if they'd be willing to show you the research proving their product can actually remove those specific toxins from your body. Chances are they won't be able to answer.

And if the cleanse is only supposed to help you lose weight, don't bother with that either. Of course you'll lose weight if you go on a weekend juice fast. Problem is, you'll gain all the weight back as soon as you start eating again.

While water isn't going to cost anywhere near as much money, it won't help you wage war on vaguely defined toxins. If you think you should detox because you feel depressed, fatigued or ill, go visit a doctor, not a health blog or a natural foods store.

10. Bottled water is better than tap water.

I love my bottled water. It's convenient. I pick it up and take it with me everywhere.

This is probably bad for the environment. I should probably use tap water. Tap water has fluoride and smart people who make the water come out of holes in my house. Tap water is so good bottled water is made from it. Without tap water, I would have to lick puddles.

There are also a lot of mental and emotional benefits to being satisfied with tap water. Let's dig into those next.

4

WATER AS SELF-HELP

Drinking extra water won't moisturize your skin, your morning coffee won't dehydrate you, and most bottled water is pumped from municipal sources, not carried to the bottling plant in the beaks of songbirds and on the tongues of baby deer.

So for the most part, the myths and old wives' tales surrounding water are misleading at best. So what hope is there for someone trying to find an intrinsic reason for drinking more water? What benefit does increasing your water consumption actually provide? As it turns out, if we dig under the surface, most of the best reasons to drink more water relate to your mental, not physical, wellbeing.

We usually think of water as a way to improve skin or lose weight or hydrate ourselves. We rarely think of the untold benefits that can be summoned from drinking water as a way to simplify our lives or strengthen our inner selves—our relationships, our emotions, our productivity. But most of us are held back further by our mindset than our bodies. If you're worried about your skin, your weight or your caffeine intake, there's a deeper reason for it.

Do you wish you had better skin? Ask yourself why. Ask yourself what you're losing by not having better skin. Ask yourself if the energy you spend thinking about your skin outweighs the benefit of solving the problem. And ask yourself why you haven't solved it already.

Do you wish you could lose weight? There are plenty of great reasons to drop pounds, but have you done the hard work and heavy lifting required to understand the real reasons driving your goal? If you've tried to lose weight before and failed, ask yourself what stood in your way. Was it that losing weight stopped being a priority, or did your mindset and situational obstacles prevent you from accomplishing your goals?

Most of the time, the things we worry about are trivial, maybe even vain. With a good enough why, we can push through almost any obstacle. And if we can't, we'll keep searching for solutions until we find one that works.

While none of the following benefits of drinking water may be big enough on their own, the profound mental shift they can provide will augment your core reason for drinking more water, whatever that happens to be. And combined, they just might make a difference in your life all on their own.

1. Be more resilient

Coffee, soda, milkshakes, and hot chocolate are luxuries. For a few dollars, we can have them whenever we want. Even bottled water and filtered water are modern conveniences that people have gone without for centuries.

We can practice resilience by drinking the most natural and easily available source of water we can find. I don't mean catching rain or boiling pond water—there's no need to go that far if you don't have to. But if the water that comes out of your tap is good enough for bathing and cooking, it's good enough for drinking. And by giving up the delicious drinks we buy at the store—even if we only choose to pass on them occasionally—we prepare ourselves for those times when luxuries aren't easy to come by.

Whether you start by replacing one drink a week with a glass of ice water or throw yourself into a 30-day challenge to drink nothing that isn't lukewarm and straight from the tap, you'll build your resilience and practice finding joy in simple things.

2. Become antifragile

Nothing's more unattractive than a whiner. Didn't have time for coffee this morning? The restaurant's out of tea or soda? No one cares, and complaining about it only makes us look bad.

It's easy to become angry or indignant or start making excuses and pointing fingers when things don't go our way, but it's never the best course of action. And when it's over little things, it's downright absurd.

When I used to drink water with lemon juice (and only with lemon juice), every time I ran out became a minor catastrophe. I'd be upset and frustrated all day. I'd blame other people for not buying more lemon juice instead of having paid enough attention to buy it myself in the first place. I was a wreck for absolutely no reason.

How do most of us react when someone else whines about something stupid? We judge them. They're either having a bad day or a bad life. Or they're just an overly critical buzzkill. We distance ourselves from them, and we definitely don't want to be like them.

So if you missed your shot of caffeine or can't get your favorite beverage, you can make yourself stronger by being happy—sincerely happy—with a simple glass of water.

A lot of people around us may fall apart. "I can't function without my coffee." "I can't believe they're out of Sprite! How do you run out of Sprite?" But we don't have to. We can adapt to the circumstances and appreciate our own strength in adapting.

3. Enjoy simple things

Building on resilience and antifragility, for those two practices to mean anything, we have to embrace water. We have to really learn to enjoy it, the same way we might appreciate a good milkshake or a finely-crafted IPA.

This can be an uphill battle if you've never liked to drink plain water. But it's a practice. When you're drinking a glass of water, focus on what's good about the water, how good it tastes and how grateful you are to live in a time and place where clean water is abundant and thirst is rare.

4. Save money

Not all the benefits have to be cerebral and tinged with self-improvement advice. Saving money is as good a reason as any other.

The cost of beverages adds up quickly. Bar tabs can be exorbitant, and the liquor store isn't much better unless you settle for bottom shelf. Coffee shops eat away a few dollars at a time, and even a big can of coffee grounds to brew at home isn't free.

Water right out of the tap is the least expensive beverage you can buy. Sticking to water can be a easy way to keep a few dollars in your pocket when money is tight. You can always splurge on calories and caffeine on special occasions or when someone else is paying.

5. Worry less

If you're conscious of your caffeine intake or calorie consumption, you may spend a lot of time thinking about it. "Ugh, there were way to many calories in that." "That was so good. I really want another...but no, I really shouldn't."

Drinking water eliminates those worries. It has zero calories and there's no caffeine or alcohol to worry about. You take a lot of mental stress off your plate when you eliminate those concerns.

This definitely isn't a cure-all for every worry, but it will rid you of a few of them and teach you how to channel some of your other worries towards productive ends and onto actions you can control.

6. Feel in control

Most of us want to feel like we're in control of our lives. We want to believe that our actions can influence the course of events. We hate feeling helpless.

If you've ever complained about the economy or the price of gas, you'll understand. Those things are outside of our immediate control. There's no specific action we can take individually to fix the economy or reduce the price of gas. To really take control in our lives, we must accept reality as it is and adapt ourselves to situations objectively. (That's easy to write, but it's by no means easy to accomplish.)

On a smaller, more personal level, imagine someone struggling with eating too much junk food. They know it's bad for them, but the compulsion is too strong. They take all the common advice like keep the snacks out of the house, but they still end up driving to the store several times a week for a bag of chips. How does this affect them? They feel awful, out of control. They're struggling against a problem they don't fully understand, a problem that breaks their willpower and crushes their sense of self-efficacy.

Just possessing that sense of control alone can help many of us. It's part of why placebos work, and it's the root of much superstitious behavior. The athlete knows his lucky socks aren't truly magic, but losing them might throw off his mental state enough that he can't compete at the highest level.

When it comes to our health, our confidence and sense of self-efficacy play a huge role. We want to be confident that we're on the right path, that what we're doing to achieve our health goals will actually get us there. This is why supplements and health foods are marketed with testimonials—their effectiveness is mostly unproven (and sometimes even disproven), but satisfied customers telling us their amazing results build our confidence in the products.

We also want to be in control, so we do things that give us that feeling, even if it's only imagined. Most of us don't need a daily multivitamin, but that one pill everyday makes us feel like we're doing something good for our bodies. And most of us aren't at a stage in our fitness journeys where we need to inhale protein shakes to meet our goals, but some of us still do; having that high-calorie protein shake or dropping a scoop of powder in a smoothie simply feels like a healthy thing to do. And in situations that are entirely out of our control, a lot of us would rather do something—anything—as long as it gives us a sense of power over the situation.

This false sense of control isn't bad. But it usually involves spending large sums of money on questionable products. On the other hand, we can feel in control of our lives—and actually take control of them—by drinking more water. While water can't make extreme health claims—builds muscle! reverses autism! cures cancer!—it provides the opportunity for us to take responsibility for our health choices. It allows us to boost our sense of self-efficacy by knowing that we chose, at least this one time, to trade a sugary, alcoholic, or caffeinated beverage for a simple glass of water.

7. Connect with nature

No, I'm not going to suggest you carry a bucket down to the nearest river. But with all the processed beverages that line grocery store shelves, water—whether bottled, filtered, or straight from the tap—is the closest a lot of us get to a natural beverage. Water, really, is the only natural beverage. So in whatever form it's available, start there, because clean water is a gift. Drink it, appreciate it, and remember that water is what nature gave us. The fact that we have an abundant supply of clean water piped directly into our homes is a testament to our ingenuity as a species.

The next time you drink water, think about that. You don't have to scoop it up with your hand or a primitive bowl. You don't even have to take the glass out side and smell the breeze. You can commune with nature from the comfort of your living room, from a cramped subway car, or while standing on stage speaking in public. All you have to do is acknowledge what a gift our easy access to water really is.

8. Free your mind for more important decisions

We make hundreds of decisions each day. From what to wear to what to eat to every time we choose to get up and walk somewhere, even if that's only to the other side of the room.

One secret of productivity is to create habits that reduce the number of decisions we have to make every day. By building habits and routines, our behaviors become automatic, and we're no longer forced to expend mental energy on small decisions. That frees our minds to focus on more important tasks.

We can also reduce our cognitive load by eliminating options and setting defaults. For example, most of us spend time choosing an outfit everyday, but others don't spend much time thinking about clothes at all. My dad wore jeans and a gray pocket tee every day for years. Recently, I've defaulted to something similar: I wear jeans and a white t-shirt almost exclusively, but I rarely even change out of my pajamas unless I'm leaving the house. I also refuse to wear shoes that need to be tied, just because I hate doing it. Tying shoes only seems to waste a minute or two, and to tell the truth I was never very good at it anyway.

But it's not only lazy people in t-shirts that do this. I've met several people who have one outfit for every day of the week and never vary from that pattern. Even Barack Obama has limited the style of suits he wears. This lack of variety in his wardrobe gives him more time to focus on the demanding work of being president.

In terms of our beverage consumption, by choosing a healthy default like water, we no longer have to think about what we're going to drink. We don't have to walk through the beverage aisle at the grocery store looking for something that catches our eyes or our taste buds. We don't have to choose from all the soda, beer, and cocktail options available at restaurants. All we have to do is build the habit of drinking water. Whenever we want a drink or feel thirsty, that should trigger us towards a glass of water and not a complex decision over the optimal way to quench our thirst.

How do we turn drinking water into a habit? That's the subject of the next chapter.

5

MAKE WATER A HABIT

I don't have a hamper. I spent the last several months building, maintaining, and tweaking a system to keep my bedroom neat and organized, but I don't have a hamper. And I do occasionally wear clothes.

I've struggled with organization most of my life, spending my childhood through my mid-twenties navigating a maze of knee-high junk and only cleaning when my mom yelled at me or I stepped on something and hurt my foot. It was, frankly, borderline hoarding, and my newly spartan room has been a revelation.

But I still don't have a hamper. There's no good, proper, government-approved place for me to store dirty clothes. But this lack of stuff has been incredibly liberating and I don't want a hamper. I don't want to sacrifice the floor space. I don't want to look at it. But after putting in all that work figuring out how to solve my organizational deficits, I refused to knuckle under and drop my clothes on the floor like I had always done.

I took a few weeks. Right after I had my room stripped bared for the first time ever, knuckle under is exactly what I did. Whenever I changed, I just tossed my clothes on the floor. But that pile ate at my mind and I would just stare at it full of confusion and resent. One day I got fed up, shoved the pile in the closet, and shut the door. It was a half-ass solution, but it eliminated the problem and lifted the fog of worry and anxiety that had been hanging around ever since I straightened the rest of my room. And every day after that, when I would get a new outfit out of the closet, I'd throw the old one in.

I can't pinpoint when I decided to do this. It never felt like a conscious decision. But now it's a habit, so much so that I did a double take the other day when I came home and saw my pajamas splayed on the bedroom floor.

And for most of us, a lot of our habits—maybe all of them—come about like this. They sneak up on us through repetition, shortcuts, and our mindless day-to-day behavior. Psychologists call humans *cognitive misers* because we're always trying to conserve mental resources. If we don't actively build habits and routines, we fall into them anyway. And the ones we fall into probably aren't the ones we want.

Our drinking habits are no different. We drink the same things we usually drink, at the same time and with the same people we usually drink them. We even hold our drinking glass in the same hand. And there's a good chance we have little clue about why we do those things.

That, in a nutshell, is habit. And escaping from the iron grip of habit requires conscious, dedicated effort to build routines and make our new behaviors automatic. It's not an easy process. You may have heard it takes 21 or 30 days to make a habit stick, but the formula isn't that simple. We have reasons for the things we do, even if we're not conscious of them. We don't always know what motivates our habits.

If you drink a Coke, a cappuccino, or a Coors Light every day, that drink fills some need for you. You may not know what it is, but it's there, and until you understand that need, you'll have limited success in changing the behavior.

To figure out what need is being fulfilled, you need to break your habits apart and examine them.

The Habit Loop:
How to pinpoint what your habits are, why they exist, and how to change them

In *The Power of Habit*, Charles Duhigg identifies a three-part habit loop that governs our behaviors.

The three parts of the habit loop are the cue, the routine, and the reward.

The cue is whatever triggers the behavior. It could be a place, a person, an action, a time of day—almost anything.

The routine is the behavior itself. This is going for that jog, opening that book, or preparing that salad. It's also hitting the snooze button, biting your nails, or devouring a second slice of cake.

The reward is what you get out of the behavior. A cup of coffee might lift your energy, give you a chance to socialize, or just be an excuse to get up and stretch your legs.

A bit of a weird personal example. I sometimes get this craving to just sit around at night listening to music. But I find it kind of boring, sitting there listening to music. And if I surf the internet at the same time, I miss the lyrics and stop paying attention to the music. But with a few beers or a couple shots of rum, I can hang out, sing along, and have a decent night. But wasting money on alcohol to drink alone listening to country songs about drinking alone isn't something I want to do on a regular basis. So I broke the habit down and found a different way to satisfy the craving.

Here's the initial habit loop:

Cue: Desire to listen to music without boredom or distractions.

Routine: Buy alcohol and have a few drinks while listening.

Reward: Enjoyed the focused listening experience.

According to Charles Duhigg, the secret to changing habits is to identify the habit loop and experiment with different routines when the cue strikes until you find another routine that provides the same reward.

For my drinking to music habit, I found that if I threw on headphones and took a walk—usually just pacing around the backyard like a weirdo for 15 to 20 minutes—I'd get the same enjoyment without spending money, wasting the whole night, or feeling like shit the next day.

You can use this same cue-routine-reward framework to identify your habits and start testing ways to change them.

Action steps for identifying and changing your beverage habits

ONE

Get a notebook, a piece of paper, or an old receipt— or open your preferred note-taking software—and write down all the beverages you drink in an average day. Mentally rehearse your day from the time you wake up to the time you go to bed and jot down everything in order from morning to night. For example, if you have coffee at 6am, 10am, and

2pm, write it down three times. If there's a drink you have everyday or almost everyday but not at any particular time, fit it in the list as best you can, even if that's just tacking it on the end.

TWO

Review your list of drinks and pick one—only one— that you'd like to change. It's easier to start small and focus on a single habit than to completely redesign your life in one go.

THREE

Identify the cue for that drink. Over the next few days or the next week, pay attention when the craving strikes and figure out exactly what triggers the behavior. Is it a person? A place? A time of day? Something else?

FOUR

Based on the cue you discovered in step three and the routine (the drink itself), brainstorm possible rewards you may get from that drink. For example, a sugary latte could be an afternoon pick-me-up, a chance to socialize, or something to satisfy your sweet tooth.

FIVE

For each possible reward, brainstorm at least one alternative routine that could replace the drink and still satisfy the reward. For example, if you always have coffee when you meet with your friends, you could order water the next time you meet with them to test the hypothesis that your reward is simply spending time with people whose company you enjoy.

SIX

Test each replacement routine until you identify the reward. Once you've identified the reward, you can build a new, healthier routine around the original cue.

6

WHEN TO DRINK MORE WATER

Some of us struggle with finding the right time to fit more water into our diets. We want to drink more water, but we enjoy the routines we already have. The morning coffee, the soda with lunch, the cocktail at the restaurant—these are simple pleasures we don't want to give up.

And a health expert rushing in wagging their finger and shouting about how bad those things are for us won't actually change our behavior. We already know soda isn't healthy. It's not a secret that lattes are packed with calories if you add in heaps of sugar and flavored syrup. So in the end, we write off the expert's advice because it's impractical. And if it sticks in the back of our mind, all it does is make us feel guilty about the things we enjoy.

So instead of admonishing you about how unhealthy everything is, I'd like to suggest six times when you can add a glass of water to your day without replacing the things you're already drinking.

1. Drink a glass of water first thing in the morning.

The easiest way to meet your hydration goals is to start the day off right. Having a glass of water right after you get out of bed will build momentum and propel you through the day.

Aside from the mental victory and the head start you get by having water at the beginning of the day, the morning is also a great time to drink a glass of water for another reason: you haven't had anything to drink in a while.

You've been sleeping for the past six to eight hours. You haven't had anything to drink in all that time, and a glass of water now will keep your body hydrated and your mind clear.

2. Drink a glass of water before each meal.

Like having a glass of water in the morning, before mealtimes is another natural place to squeeze extra water into your day. If you're cooking for yourself, drink a glass of water while preparing your meal. If someone else is cooking, finish a glass of water before sitting down to eat.

3. Drink water before, during, and after exercise.

Unless you live underwater, it's no secret you sweat when you exercise. So the best way to keep hydrated during exercise is to be well hydrated when you start and to keep up your water intake as you get moving.

Make sure you've had water recently before starting your workout, and keep a big bottle of water at hand until you've finished, taking a sip or a glug as often as you need.

And when you're finished working out, that's an excellent time to rehydrate. I always drink a half-liter bottle of water immediately after I finish any sort of exercise, even if it's just a ten-minute walk.

4. Match every alcoholic drink with a glass of water.

A clever wino faces a spectacular opportunity to boost his water intake with this tip. And if you aren't a wino, or are in denial about being a wino, you still might get some mileage out of it.

There are several benefits to drinking a glass of water after every alcoholic beverage you enjoy. The water will keep you sober longer by slowing down your alcohol intake. The increased water intake while drinking also makes the morning after a whole lot easier. Dehydration is a significant cause of hangovers, and pacing yourself drink for drink with a glass of water will ease or eliminate that shitty feeling the next day.

5. Drink a full glass of water when taking medications or vitamins.

A lot of medications, vitamins, and supplements are meant to be taken with water. It usually says so on the bottle. But check first. I'm not your doctor.

If your pills are okay to take with water, polish off a full glass when you wash them down. This is one of my favorite tactics because it stacks right on top of a routine many of us already have.

6. Drink a glass of water after every coffee, tea, juice, or soda.

Instead of denying yourself beverages that you enjoy, used them to set up good habits. When you choose to drink coffee, tea, juice or soda, you can also choose what to do when you finish the drink. This is the perfect time to set up a new habit, because finishing the drink acts as a trigger.

You can formulate your habit as follows: *After I finish a soda, I will drink a glass of water.*

Then when you finish the water smile to yourself or celebrate out loud to help cement the habit with a small reward.

Those are six simple and common places to squeeze more water into your day. Just on of them could significantly boost your water intake. And almost everyone can find at least one of the six that works for them.

But there are other ways to fit more water into your day. In the next chapter, I discuss two tactics for making water a part of your daily life.

7

MAKE WATER PART OF YOUR DAILY LIFE

Aside from building habits around drinking water at specific times, it's also a good idea to build access to water into your daily life. In the modern world, there's no reason for most of us to be too far from clean water at any time. But if you often catch yourself out of the house without something to drink or reaching for a soda just because the bottle's in the fridge, these two tactics will help you make water part of your daily life, if not your go-to beverage.

1. Carry water with you wherever you go.

Taking water with you wherever you go is a great habit to get into. If you're trying to increase your water intake, having water nearby at all times is a great way to reduce the friction between wanting to drink more water and actually doing it. It's much easier to reach across your desk than it is to get up and walk to across the room.

Research has shown that moving a bowl of chocolates off the desk and six feet across the room will discourage us from eating sweets. We're even prone to eating less chocolate if the bowl is just hidden away in a drawer or made of an opaque material instead of clear glass. Not being able to see the chocolate reduces the temptation. And our natural laziness as a species keeps us from taking three steps to grab a Hershey's Kiss.

But in the case of water, more is a good thing. So keep your water bottle in sight, at hand, and always available.

2. Don't keep other drinks in the house.

A simple way to force yourself to drink more water is to keep other drinks out of the house. Like with any junk food, just the presence of sweetened beverages increases the chance you'll drink them. In fact, it almost guarantees it.

If your house is full of unhealthy drinks, throw them out or finish them off and don't buy more. Limit the beverages you keep at home to water and other healthy staples like black coffee and herbal tea.

This tactic will unquestionably reduce your consumption of unhealthy drinks, but it's also pretty extreme for a lot of people. If you want to cut back on junk without taking such drastic measures, I share several tactics you can use to make healthier beverage choices in the next chapter.

8

DRINK LESS OF EVERYTHING ELSE

When we decide to drink more water, often it's because we know our current beverage choices aren't the best for us. And when that's the case, finding ways to cut down on the unhealthy beverages we're drinking can make all the difference.

None of the following tactics are the result of groundbreaking research. They're all common sense tips you've probably heard before. But if you're not putting them into practice already, hopefully collecting them all here will jog your memory and get you in motion. Combined with the cue-routine-reward framework for building habits, some oft-ignored common sense advice becomes much easier to follow.

1. Replace sugary drinks.

You can fit more water into your day by replacing what you're already drinking. To get started, go through your day to figure out what you're drinking and when. Write down a list of all the different beverages you consume. Next, decide which of those beverages you can most easily switch out for water. You may not want to give up all your other drinks, but getting rid of one or two can boost your water intake and improve your health all in one go. Here's why:

Most drinks besides water are laden with sugar and calories. Soda is sugar and calories, fruit juice is sugar and calories, alcohol is sugar and calories—hell, milk is mostly sugar and calories. Replacing a single one of those drinks with a glass of water will slash 100 to 200 empty calories from your day and lead to effortless weight loss.

2. Replace caffeinated drinks.

The few beverages that don't contain a bunch of calories are usually loaded with caffeine. While coffee and tea are fine in moderation, when they become a daily ritual, your body adjusts and you may not get as much of a boost as you used to. If you're using modest amounts of caffeine to enhance your productivity—and it's working—by all means keep it up. But if caffeine's just a habit—that cup of coffee nothing more than a social event, that afternoon tea only a reason to lift up your pinky and look down your nose—consider swapping in a glass of water.

If coffee and tea are social events, remember that you make the rules. Just like you can order water at the bar instead of a pitcher of Long Island Iced Tea, the barista at Starbuck's isn't secretly judging you for not ordering a latte. Well, maybe she is, but you can comfort yourself with the knowledge that she has a master's degree, $30,000 in student loan debt, and neither the hard skills nor the social skills to become a stripper.

And if the friends and coworkers you drink coffee with are judging you, punch them in the dick.

3. Read the labels on flavored water.

I feel like an ass for giving this advice. Nutrition experts harping on how you should read the labels on products annoy the hell out of me. Most of us with a bit of interest in diet and health already know about nutrition labels. I don't think I've ever met someone who didn't know about them. Sure, there are plenty of people who don't care what's in their food, but even they know the labels exist. So I really hate even mentioning this.

But it's important, because flavored water is actually a notorious hellhole for hidden sugar and calories. While San Pellegrino's sparkling mineral water is calorie free, the flavored versions contain over 30 grams of sugar—almost as much as Coke or Mountain Dew.

And don't get me started on Vitaminwater. Vitaminwater is water in the same way that ketchup is a vegetable.

4. Buy unhealthy drinks in small bottles.

I recently realized Ben & Jerry's sells little baby single serve ice cream cups. And I wanted some ice cream, but not very much. So instead of buying a pint of Cherry Garcia, I snagged two four-ounce containers. What happened is I ate half as much ice cream as I would have if I bought the pint, and I still satisfied my craving to have a bit of ice cream this summer.

You can do the same thing with sugary beverages. It's not a moral failing to drink Coke, but it's also not a good way to treat your body on a regular basis. So when you want soda or pomegranate juice or Red Bull or Yoo-hoo, buy the smallest option available.

A single serving you'll finish in one go is best, but sometimes you'll have to buy more than that. If that's the case, a six-pack is better than a two-liter bottle, because the amount you can drink at once is limited. If you want more, you have to open another can. And that pause point where you have to stop and open another can means you have to think about what you're doing. And that's the important part: We want to be making conscious decisions, not following mindless impulses. We don't have to make perfect decisions every time, but we do owe it to ourselves to be mindful of our behavior.

5. Be the designated driver.

You can cut down on your calorie and alcohol intake by volunteering to be designated driver when your friends go out drinking. You empower yourself by choosing to not drink and taking charge of your health for the night. You also help your friends get home safe.

Some people have hang-ups about not drinking when everyone else is. People may repeatedly offer you drinks, ask why you don't drink, stare in utter disbelief when you continue to refuse, and wonder if you're a recovering alcoholic. Ignore those people. You don't have to drink.

If you tell them you're playing designated driver, they may nudge you to have just one or two. You don't have to do that either. No is a wonderful word. Use it more.

6. Order healthy drinks when eating out.

A restaurant is the best place to screw up your diet. I always forget my heath at restaurants. It's more fun that way. I don't want to worry about calories or carbs or trans fats when I go out to eat.

But I always drink iced tea at restaurants. No sugar. That's what I always drink at home too.

But some people aren't me. Maybe they like deciding which $15 salad is the least worst. And maybe they drink lots of soda and alcohol at restaurants. So they need to be told, hey, have some water.

If that's you, have some water next time you go out to dinner. Or unsweetened tea. I prefer tea.

7. Use tall, thin glasses for unhealthy beverages.

This is a weird tip based on psychology research and visual illusions. It turns out, short and wide glasses cause even experienced bartenders to over-pour drinks. Because tall and thin glasses give the illusion of more volume, we pour less.

To use this to our advantage, serve beverages you want to drink less of in tall, thin glasses. You'll pour less and drink less without even noticing.

If we combine these tactics for cutting back with the earlier advice on drinking more water, creating a healthier relationship with the beverages we drink becomes inevitable. But to make sure the these new behaviors fit into your life seamlessly and stick for years to come, we need to know how to track our water intake so we can celebrate victories and correct course if we start to drift off target. In the next chapter, I share my favorite methods and tools for tracking both daily and long-term water intake.

9

HOW TO TRACK YOUR WATER INTAKE

Depending on your goals, you won't necessarily need to track your water intake. In fact, if you increase your water intake by building habits around it—always having a glass first thing in the morning, always drinking a full glass when you take medications or vitamins, having water before every meal—there may not be any need to track what you're doing. If you default to water when you want a drink, tracking your intake with even the simplest system is overkill.

But if your water intake isn't slotted into your daily routine—and it probably won't be at first—measuring how much water you're actually drinking can help you guarantee you're hitting your goals. And if you're falling behind, having the data available allows you to diagnose when, where, and how it went wrong.

When you track your water intake, there are two different metrics you may want to track. First, you can track your daily water intake. If you want to drink 64oz of water a day, you're probably not going to do it all at once, so you need a tool that allows you to break your daily intake down by cups, ounces, liters, or whatever becomes your preferred serving size. Second, you may want to track your long-term water intake. That is, how many days in a row did you hit your goal.

Both of these can be tracked with nothing more than paper and pen. Most of the time, that's the option I prefer myself. But you may like other tools, especially if you spend more time with a cell phone than a notebook in your hands. It would be impossible to include an exhaustive list of apps that track water intake, so in the list below I've included only those I've used personally.

How to track your daily water intake on paper

When tracking your daily water intake, all you need to do is break your goal into discreet chunks and make a note when you complete one of those chunks. For example, if you want to drink eight eight-ounce glasses of water a day, you'll make a check every time you drink a cup of water.

For tracking water intake, my definition of paper is broad. In the past, I've tracked different goals and habits with a variety of things. The only important point is to grab something you don't mind scarring with a pen.

SCRAP PAPER

This is the most temporary and haphazard option of all, the equivalent of sketching up your business idea on the back of a napkin. In fact, a napkin serves the same trick. Grab a loose receipt, a napkin, or scrap torn off a junk mail envelope and draw a tick mark for every glass of water you drink. You can even stuff the receipt in your pocket and carry it with you through the day so you're never without it. This method is disposable by design, but if you use different areas of the paper, one receipt can last several days.

INDEX & BUSINESS CARDS

For a while, this was my favorite option. I would draw boxes on index cards or blank-backed business cards and stick them to my bedroom door with Blu-Tack. Then when I drank a bottle of water, I'd X off a box. Depending on the size of the card and how many times a day you want to drink water, a single card can fit enough boxes to last a week or possibly even a month.

NOTEBOOKS

This is the option I'm using now. Every day I turn to a new page in my notebook and, at the top of the page, just above the first line, I write the date. Then I skip a line and write down my three most important tasks for the day. On that skipped line, I draw an X each time I finish a bottle of water. (When I started, I drew little cups and colored them in. That didn't last long.)

How to track your daily water intake with an app

Using an app to track water intake isn't my preferred solution because paper has always seemed easier. However, here are three apps I've tested and used for other purposes. They're all free, and I'm satisfied with how well each of them work.

MYFITNESSPAL (web, Android, and iOS, free)

There are many apps that let you log your meals and track your calories, but I've always preferred MyFitnessPal because of its large food database. It also allows you to log how many cups of water you drink each day. If you're logging your food anyway, keeping track of your water intake while logging your meals could be an easy solution.

FITBIT (web, Android, and iOS, free)

Similar to MyFitnessPal, the Fitbit app allows you to track your water intake. You don't need to own a Fitbit activity tracker to use the app, but I don't see why you'd choose it if you don't. I love—absolutely love—my Fitbit, but I wouldn't use the app to manually track anything. But if you have a Fitbit and only want one health app on your phone or tablet, Fitbit's app lets you input your daily cups of water.

STRIDES (web and iOS, free)

Strides is an app that lets you track habits and goals. It can do a lot, and for me that's its biggest downside. But you might love it and find multiple uses for it beyond just tracking water. If you only want to track your water intake, you could use it to set a single goal of drinking your preferred amount of water each day.

How to track your long-term water intake on paper

Jerry Seinfeld's advice on how he writes jokes every day has become a classic productivity tip: He got a calendar and drew a big red X through each day he wrote a joke. Eventually he built up a chain of X's and kept going because he didn't want to break the chain. That's essentially the goal with tracking long-term water intake as well: Mark off every day you hit your goal and don't break the chain.

For long-term habits, I've come to prefer using an app. But if you'd like to keep track of yours on paper, here are a few of the best options.

INDEX CARDS, BUSINESS CARDS & NOTEBOOKS

To measure your streak and start building your chain using paper, simply draw boxes representing each day and check one off every time you accomplish your daily goal. I've found I can squeeze enough boxes on the back of a business card to cover a whole month, so with this compact system you could fit an entire year's habit chain on one page of a notebook.

CALENDARS

Seinfeld's classic calendar method is great for accountability if you have a calendar already hanging on your wall. Starting today, every time you complete your goal, draw a big X through the date with a red marker. Don't break the chain.

How to track long-term
water intake with an app

The index cards I used to track long-term habits and goals began to clutter up my wall and I wanted to get rid of them. So I began testing apps to see which ones worked best to keep me on track and keep my habit streaks going. Neither of these options work with Android devices, but a quick Google search tells me there are plenty of choices available. I didn't want to include anything I couldn't personally vouch for.

HABIT LIST (iOS only, $3.99)

I first heard this app mentioned by Chase Jarvis in an interview he did with James Altucher. The app appears minimalist but is deceptively powerful. It's designed entirely to record your chain of daily habits. It also able to lets you set up habits you only want to do a set number of times a week or only on certain days. This is my current solution for long-term, don't-break-the-chain goals, and I'd happily spend the $4 again.

STRIDES (web and iOS, free)

Strides can not only help track your daily water intake but can also keep a running streak of days when you hit your goal. Strides is a wonderful all-around solution for tracking habits and goals, and the only reason I don't use it is because it's overkill for my needs.

Now that we have the tools we need to track our water intake, I'm going wrap everything back up in the **O.A.S.I.S.** framework and show you how to build your new water habits with a system that works like a well-oiled machine.

Onward.

10

O.A.S.I.S. IN ACTION

Now, as the train pulls into the station and the passengers disembark, it's time for one final round-up of all we've covered on our journey, one last walk through the **O.A.S.I.S. Method** so you can see how it applies to the strategies outlined in the book.

1. OVERCOME obstacles and myths

We studied the common mental barriers that hold us back from our hydration goals and injected some sense into the dubious claims that circulate around water. We learned that what holds us back is often not external pressures but our mindsets and limiting beliefs.

If you don't like the taste of water, that can be overcome with filters, flavoring or—if you're bold—

sheer force of will. If the price of bottled or filtered water is an issue, that too can be overcome; tap water is an amazing resource, and since you have to drink something unless you plan to die of thirst, price can never be an excuse.

We learned that our water needs vary from person to person and that both our food and other beverages count towards our water intake goals. In Chapter 4, we also discovered eight unconventional ways water can improve our lives, from increasing our resilience and reducing our worries to augmenting our sense of self-efficacy and helping us save money.

2. ACKNOWLEDGE current habits

In Chapter 5, we got brutally honest with ourselves. After understanding the cue-routine-reward framework of the habit loop, we dug into our current routines and relationships with water and other beverages and devised experiments to help us change them.

3. START changing bad habits

Here's where we identified and tested small changes to see which could fit into our lives for the long term. Not only did we look at ways to fit water into our lives and take out less desirable choices, we also learned the power of common-sense advice when put into action.

4. INCREASE water intake

As we moved forward, we discussed several tactics and lifestyle changes that could help us increase our water intake. From adding water to our current routines to carrying water with us everywhere we go, we considered a range of options that could fit comfortably into any lifestyle.

5. STUDY the results

And finally, with our destination in sight, I shared my favorite methods and tools for tracking daily and long-term water intake. Once you've been tracking for a few weeks, it's time to study the data and find out how your new habits are working.

If they're not, study the times when you missed your goals and find the patterns that bind them together. Then, empowered by the information you've collected, tweak your habits until you find a combination that's sustainable in the long term.

But if they are working, celebrate your victory and keep chugging along. Or better yet, use your newfound knowledge of habit creation and the momentum of success improve even more areas of your life.

On the next page, in Chapter 11, I've summed up the entire premise of this book in seven words. And that's where our journey together ends, with those seven words. See you there.

11

SEVEN WORD SUMMARY

Find water. Put it in your mouth.

BEFORE YOU **GO...**

I really appreciate you taking the time to read this book. If you take just one idea and use it to improve your life, I'll have accomplished what I set out to do.

So if you made it this far and enjoyed the book, it would mean the world if you could take a short moment out of your day to post a review on Amazon. Your feedback encourages me to keep going and guides my writing towards topics my readers care about.

And whether you plan to keep this book bedside like a religious text or burn it like a competing holy book, if you're that passionate about it, I'd love to hear from you. My email address is on the next page.

CONTACT THE AUTHOR

Thanks for making it to the end of the book. Whether you loved it or hated it, read every page or skipped right to the back, I really appreciate hearing from readers. If you have questions, comments, feedback or suggestions, send me an email at esfoster@gmail.com.

GET MY EBOOK *5 FAST FLAVORED WATER RECIPES* FOR FREE

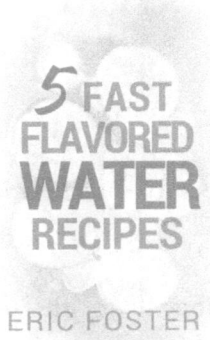

INCLUDES...

- A quick start guide of tools and techniques for making delicious flavored water

- Recipes for five exclusive blends including Citrus Sunrise, Summer Siesta Water, and Liquid Alarm Clock

- My must-have shopping list for experimenting with your own flavored water creations

DOWNLOAD NOW AT
WWW.ESFOSTER.COM/5FASTWATERS